THE ULTIMATE
OSTEOPOROSIS
DIET COOKBOOK
For Seniors

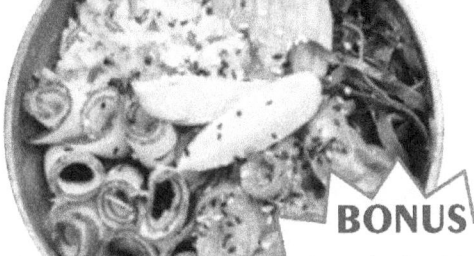

The Comprehensive Guide To Nutritious Recipes, Meal Plan, And Promote Bone Health For Seniors

BONUS

14 Weeks Meal Planner Plus 10 Healthy Exercise For Better Bone

LEONA BUTLER

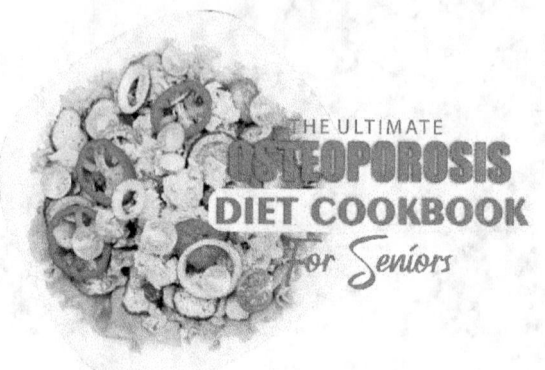

1. Gather Ingredients: Start by reviewing the recipes in the cookbook and making a list of ingredients you'll need.

2. Understand Dietary Recommendations: Familiarize yourself with the dietary recommendations for osteoporosis, such as calcium-rich foods, vitamin D sources, and foods low in sodium.

3. Plan Meals: Plan your meals for the week using the recipes in the cookbook. Aim for a variety of calcium-rich foods like dairy, leafy greens, and fortified foods.

4. Read Instructions Carefully: Before you begin cooking, read the recipe instructions carefully to ensure you understand each step.

5. Follow Portion Sizes: Pay attention to portion sizes recommended in the recipes, as overeating can lead to weight gain, which can strain bones.

6. Use Substitutions if Necessary: If you have dietary restrictions or preferences, feel free to substitute ingredients as needed while still adhering to osteoporosis-friendly guidelines.

7. Cook with Osteoporosis-Friendly Techniques: Opt for cooking methods that preserve nutrients, such as steaming vegetables or grilling lean meats.

8. Experiment with Flavors: Don't be afraid to experiment with herbs and spices to enhance flavor without adding extra salt.

9. Enjoy Balanced Meals: Once your meals are ready, sit down and enjoy them, knowing that you're nourishing your body with foods that support bone health.

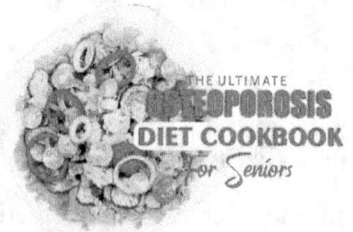

Table of content

Introduction

Chapter 1

UNDERSTANDING OSTEOPOROSIS:

IMPORTANCE OF NUTRITION IN OSTEOPOROSIS PREVENTION:

Chapter 2

THE OSTEOPOROSIS DIET: PRINCIPLES AND GUIDELINES

BUILDING A BALANCED PLATE:

FOODS TO LIMIT OR AVOID:

MEAL PLANNING STRATEGIES FOR BONE HEALTH:

Chapter 3

Breakfast Recipes For Bone Health:

1. GREEK YOGURT PARFAIT WITH MIXED BERRIES AND ALMOND SLICES:

2. SPINACH AND FETA OMELETTE WITH WHOLE GRAIN TOAST:

3. OVERNIGHT OATS WITH CHIA SEEDS, CHOPPED NUTS, AND DRIED APRICOTS:

4. AVOCADO TOAST WITH SMOKED SALMON AND POACHED EGG

5. WHOLE GRAIN PANCAKES WITH MASHED BANANA AND WALNUTS

6. KALE, PINEAPPLE, GREEK YOGURT, AND HEMP SEED SMOOTHIE

7. QUINOA BREAKFAST BOWL WITH SAUTÉED SPINACH, TOMATOES, AND A POACHED EGG:

8. COTTAGE CHEESE AND FRUIT BOWL WITH SLICED ALMONDS AND A DRIZZLE OF HONEY:

9. VEGETABLE FRITTATA WITH SWEET POTATO HASH BROWNS:

5. STUFFED ACORN SQUASH WITH GROUND TURKEY, QUINOA, AND CRANBERRIES:

6. VEGETABLE LASAGNA MADE WITH WHOLE WHEAT NOODLES AND RICOTTA CHEESE:

7. BAKED CHICKEN BREAST WITH SWEET POTATO MASH AND STEAMED GREEN BEANS

8. LENTIL AND VEGETABLE STEW SERVED WITH A SIDE OF WHOLE GRAIN BREAD

9. SHRIMP AND VEGETABLE STIR-FRY WITH SESAME GINGER SAUCE OVER BROWN RICE NOODLES

10. ROASTED CAULIFLOWER STEAKS WITH TAHINI SAUCE AND A SIDE OF WILD RICE PILAF

Chapter 6: Snacks And Desserts For Bone Support:

1. ALMOND BUTTER AND BANANA SLICES ON WHOLE GRAIN CRACKERS

2. GREEK YOGURT WITH HONEY AND SLICED ALMONDS

3. APPLE SLICES WITH ALMOND BUTTER AND CINNAMON

4. CARROT AND HUMMUS SNACK PACKS

5. TRAIL MIX WITH ALMONDS, DRIED CRANBERRIES, AND PUMPKIN SEEDS:

6. COTTAGE CHEESE WITH PINEAPPLE CHUNKS AND SUNFLOWER SEEDS

7. DARK CHOCOLATE COVERED STRAWBERRIES:

8. BAKED APPLE CHIPS SPRINKLED WITH CINNAMON:

9. CHIA SEED PUDDING WITH MIXED BERRIES

10. FROZEN YOGURT BARK WITH CHOPPED NUTS AND DRIED FRUIT

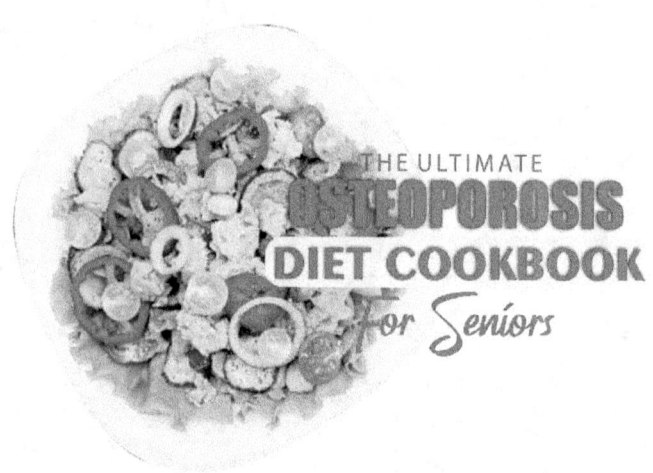

Introduction

Introducing "Bone Health Delights: An Osteoporosis Diet Cookbook for Seniors" – your essential guide to nourishing your bones and enhancing your overall well-being. In this comprehensive cookbook, we've curated a collection of delicious recipes specifically crafted to support bone health in seniors.

Packed with nutrient-rich ingredients like calcium, vitamin D, and bone-friendly foods, each recipe is carefully designed to promote strong and resilient bones while tantalizing your taste buds.

Inside, you'll find a wealth of culinary inspiration, from savory entrees to satisfying snacks, all tailored to meet the unique nutritional needs of seniors. Our recipes not only prioritize bone-strengthening nutrients but also focus on promoting healthy eating habits that can enhance your quality of life.

By incorporating these recipes into your daily routine, you'll not only reduce your risk of fractures but also enjoy improved energy levels, mood, and vitality.

But "Bone Health Delights" is more than just a cookbook – it's a comprehensive resource that empowers you to take control of your bone health. With educational resources, meal planning tips, and tailored dietary guidance, this book equips you with the knowledge and tools you need to support your long-term bone health journey.

Say goodbye to bland and boring meals – with "Bone Health Delights," you'll discover a world of flavorful, nutritious, and bone-loving dishes that will nourish your body and delight your senses.

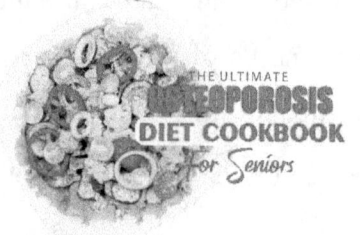

Chapter 1

Understanding Osteoporosis:

Osteoporosis, often referred to as the "silent disease," is a condition characterized by weakened bones, making them more susceptible to fractures. Despite its prevalence and significant impact on quality of life, osteoporosis is often misunderstood and underestimated. In this section, we explore the underlying causes of osteoporosis, including hormonal changes, lifestyle factors, and genetic predispositions.

We delve into the physiology of bone remodeling, highlighting the delicate balance between bone formation and resorption, and how disturbances in this balance can lead to bone loss. Through clear explanations and illustrative diagrams, readers will gain a deeper understanding of bone structure, bone density measurements, and the progression of osteoporosis.

Furthermore, we address the risk factors associated with osteoporosis, including age, gender, family history, hormonal imbalances, inadequate physical activity, smoking, excessive alcohol consumption, and poor nutrition. Understanding these risk factors is crucial for early detection, prevention, and management of osteoporosis.

Importance of Nutrition in Osteoporosis Prevention:

Nutrition plays a pivotal role in maintaining optimal bone health and preventing osteoporosis. In this section, we explore the essential nutrients necessary for building and maintaining strong bones, including calcium, vitamin D, vitamin K, magnesium, phosphorus, and protein. We provide practical guidance on incorporating these nutrients into a balanced diet and discuss the importance of supplementation when necessary.

Moreover, we delve into the impact of dietary factors such as excessive sodium intake, caffeine consumption, and acidic diets on bone health. By understanding the interplay between nutrition and bone metabolism, readers will learn how to make informed dietary choices to support their bone health goals.

Additionally, we address the importance of weight-bearing exercises and resistance training in promoting bone density and strength. Through evidence-based recommendations and practical tips, readers will discover effective strategies to integrate exercise into their daily routine for optimal bone health.

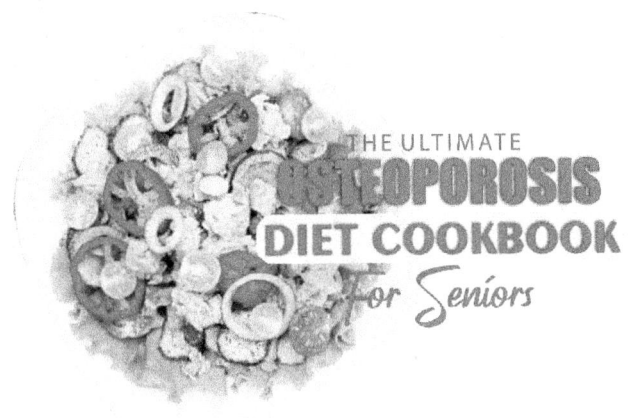

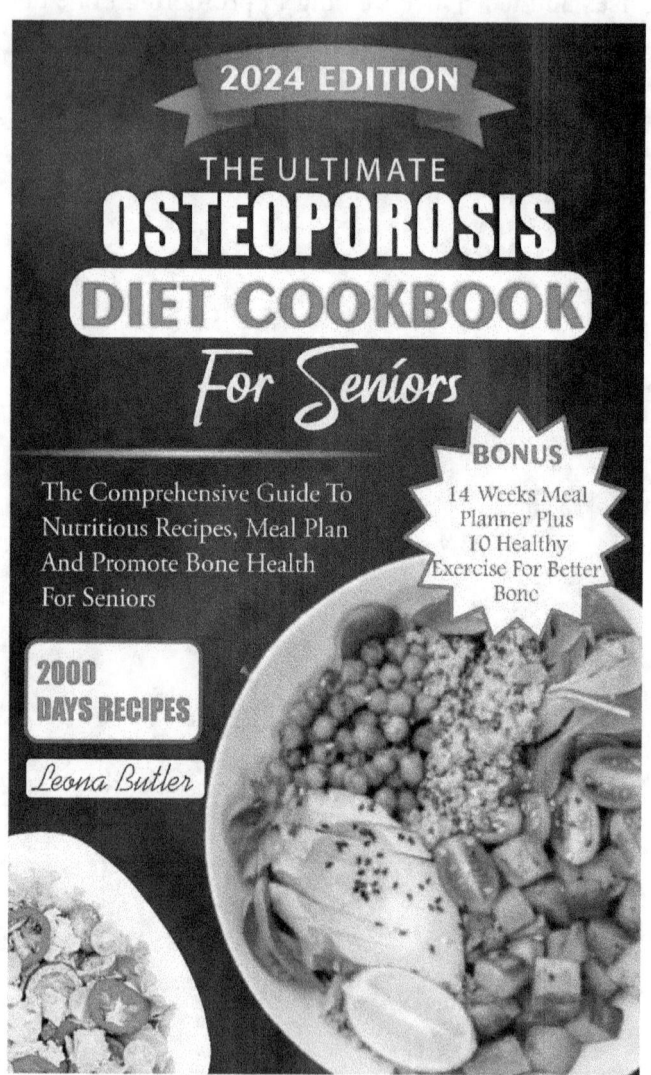

2024 EDITION

THE ULTIMATE

OSTEOPOROSIS

DIET COOKBOOK

For Seniors

The Comprehensive Guide To
Nutritious Recipes, Meal Plan
And Promote Bone Health
For Seniors

BONUS
14 Weeks Meal
Planner Plus
10 Healthy
Exercise For Better
Bone

2000 DAYS RECIPES

Leona Butler

Chapter 2

The Osteoporosis Diet: Principles and Guidelines

Osteoporosis is a condition characterized by weakened bones, making them more prone to fractures and breaks. While medications can help manage osteoporosis, diet plays a crucial role in maintaining bone health. The following principles and guidelines are essential for crafting an osteoporosis-friendly diet.

Building a Balanced Plate:

A balanced plate for osteoporosis includes foods rich in calcium, vitamin D, protein, and other nutrients essential for bone health. Calcium is a cornerstone nutrient, found in dairy products like milk, yogurt, and cheese, as well as in leafy greens like kale and broccoli.

Vitamin D aids in calcium absorption and can be obtained from sunlight exposure, fatty fish, fortified dairy products, and supplements. Protein is vital for bone strength, found in sources such as lean meats, poultry, fish, beans, and nuts. Incorporating a variety of fruits and vegetables provides antioxidants and other micronutrients beneficial for overall health.

Foods to Limit or Avoid:

Certain foods and beverages can hinder calcium absorption or contribute to bone loss, making them important to limit or avoid. High-sodium foods, such as processed snacks and canned soups, can increase calcium excretion in the urine. Excessive caffeine and alcohol intake may interfere with calcium absorption and decrease bone density. Foods high in added sugars and unhealthy fats should also be limited, as they can contribute to inflammation and compromise bone health.

Meal Planning Strategies for Bone Health:

Meal planning is key to ensuring a diet that supports bone health. Aim for three balanced meals per day, incorporating calcium-rich foods, lean proteins, and plenty of fruits and vegetables. Snacks can also contribute to nutrient intake, such as yogurt with fruit, cheese with whole-grain crackers, or nuts with dried fruit. Including a source of vitamin D in meals, such as fortified dairy or fatty fish, helps optimize calcium absorption. Consider consulting with a registered dietitian for personalized meal planning guidance tailored to individual nutritional needs and preferences.

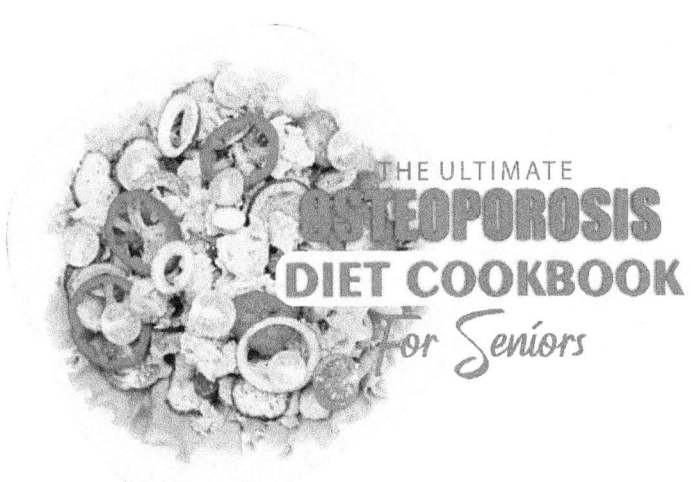

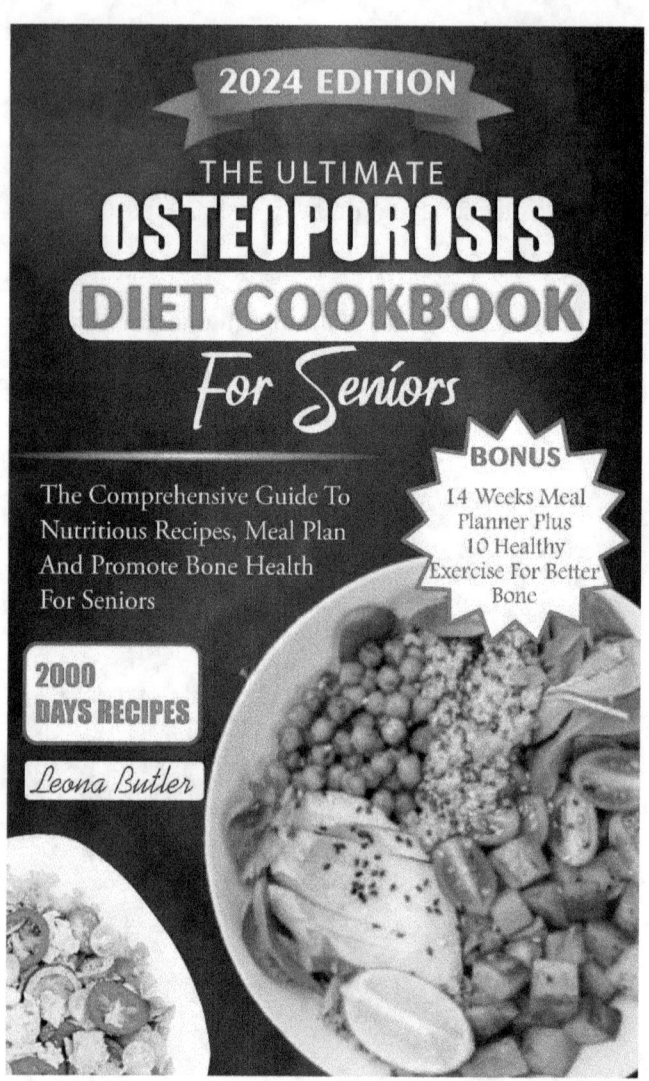

2024 EDITION

THE ULTIMATE

OSTEOPOROSIS

DIET COOKBOOK

For Seniors

The Comprehensive Guide To
Nutritious Recipes, Meal Plan
And Promote Bone Health
For Seniors

BONUS

14 Weeks Meal
Planner Plus
10 Healthy
Exercise For Better
Bone

**2000
DAYS RECIPES**

Leona Butler

Chapter 3

Breakfast Recipes for Bone Health:

1. Greek Yogurt Parfait with Mixed Berries and Almond Slices:

Ingredients:

- cup Greek yogurt
- 1/2 cup mixed berries (such strawberries, blueberries, and raspberries)
- tablespoons almond slices
- Honey or maple syrup (optional, for sweetness)

Preparation:

1. In a glass or bowl, layer Greek yogurt, mixed berries, and almond slices.
2. Drizzle honey or maple syrup for sweetness, if desired.
3. Serve immediately.

Nutritional Value:

- This parfait provides a good source of protein from the Greek yogurt and healthy fats from the almond slices.
- It's also rich in antioxidants and vitamins from the mixed berries.

Cooking Time:

Prep time: 5 minutes

2. Spinach and Feta Omelette with Whole Grain Toast:

Ingredients:

- 2 large eggs
- cup fresh spinach, chopped
- 1/4 cup crumbled feta cheese
- slices whole grain bread Salt and pepper to taste

Preparation:

1. In a bowl, whisk the eggs and season with salt and pepper.
2. Heat a non-stick skillet over medium heat and lightly coat with cooking spray or olive oil.
3. Pour the beaten eggs into the skillet.
4. Once the edges start to set, add the chopped spinach and crumbled feta cheese on one half of the omelette.
5. Fold the other half of the omelette over the filling and cook until the eggs are fully set.
6. Toast the whole grain bread slices.
7. Serve the omelette with toasted whole grain bread.

Cooking Time:

Prep time: 5 minutes

Cooking time: 5-7 minutes

3. Overnight Oats with Chia Seeds, Chopped Nuts, and Dried Apricots:

Ingredients:

- 1/2 cup rolled oats
- tablespoon chia seeds
- tablespoons of chopped nuts (such as almonds, walnuts, or pecans).
- 2 tablespoons dried apricots, chopped
- 1/2 cup milk (dairy or plant-based)
- Honey or maple syrup (optional, for sweetness)

Preparation:

1. In a jar or bowl, combine rolled oats, chia seeds, chopped nuts, and dried apricots. Pour in the milk and mix until thoroughly blended.
2. Cover the jar or bowl and refrigerate overnight.
3. In the morning, stir the oats mixture and add honey or maple syrup for sweetness, if desired. Serve cold or warm it up in the microwave before serving.

Nutritional Value:

- This overnight oats dish is packed with fiber from the oats and chia seeds, protein from the nuts, and vitamins from the dried apricots.

Cooking Time:

Prep time: 5 minutes (plus overnight refrigeration)

Cooking time: None

4. Avocado Toast with Smoked Salmon and Poached Egg

Ingredients:

- 2 slices of whole grain bread
- ripe avocado
- 100g smoked salmon
- eggs
- Salt and pepper to taste

Cooking Time: Approximately 10 minutes.

Preparation:

1. Avocado Mash: Peel and pit the avocado, then mash it in a bowl with a fork. Season with salt and pepper to taste.
2. Poached eggs: Heat a pot of water to a medium simmer. Crack the eggs into individual tiny dishes or ramekins. Gently place the eggs in the cooking water. Cook for 3-4 minutes, until the whites are set but the yolks remain liquid.
3. Toast: Toast the whole grain bread slices until golden brown.
4. Assembly: Spread the mashed avocado evenly on the toasted bread slices. Top with slices of smoked salmon.
5. Poached Eggs: Carefully remove the poached eggs from the water with a slotted spoon and place one on each avocado toast.
6. Season: Season with additional salt and pepper if desired.

Nutritional Value: Avocado provides healthy fats and fiber, salmon offers omega-3 fatty acids and protein, eggs contribute additional protein and essential vitamins.

5. Whole Grain Pancakes with Mashed Banana and Walnuts

Ingredients:

- 1 cup whole grain pancake mix
- 1 ripe banana, mashed
- 1/4 cup chopped walnuts
- 1 cup milk (or non-dairy milk alternative)
- 1 egg
- Cooking spray or butter for cooking

Preparation:

1. Mix Batter: In a mixing bowl, combine the whole grain pancake mix, mashed banana, chopped walnuts, milk, and egg. Stir until just combined.
2. Heat Pan: Heat a non-stick skillet or griddle over medium heat and lightly grease with cooking spray or butter.
3. Cook Pancakes: Pour 1/4 cup of batter onto the skillet for each pancake. Cook until bubbles appear on the surface,

then flip and continue cooking until golden brown on both sides.

4. Serve: Stack the pancakes on a plate and top with additional mashed banana and chopped walnuts if desired.

Nutritional Value: Whole grain pancakes offer fiber and complex carbohydrates, banana provides potassium and natural sweetness, walnuts add healthy fats and protein. Cooking Time: Approximately 15 minutes.

6. Kale, Pineapple, Greek Yogurt, and Hemp Seed Smoothie

Ingredients:

1. 1 cup kale leaves, stemmed and chopped
2. 1 cup frozen pineapple chunks
3. 1/2 cup Greek yogurt
4. 1 tablespoon hemp seeds
5. 1/2 cup water or unsweetened almond milk

Preparation:

1. Blend: In a blender, combine the kale leaves, frozen pineapple chunks, Greek yogurt, hemp seeds, and water or almond milk.
2. Blend Until Smooth: Blend until smooth and creamy, adding more liquid if necessary to reach your desired consistency.
3. Pour the smoothie into cups and drink immediately.

Nutritional Value: Kale provides vitamins and minerals, pineapple adds natural sweetness and vitamin C, Greek yogurt offers protein and probiotics, hemp seeds contribute omega-3 fatty acids and protein.

Cooking Time: Approximately 5 minutes.

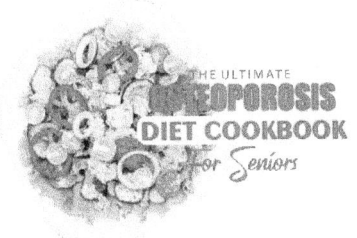

7. Quinoa breakfast bowl with sautéed spinach, tomatoes, and a poached egg:

Ingredients:

- 1/2 cup quinoa
- 1 cup water or vegetable broth
- 1 cup spinach, chopped
- 1/2 cup cherry tomatoes, halved
- 1 egg
- Salt and pepper to taste

Preparation:

1. Rinse the quinoa under cold water.
2. In a small pot, bring water or vegetable broth to a boil and add quinoa. Reduce heat, cover, and simmer for about 15 minutes or until the quinoa is cooked and the liquid is absorbed.
3. In a skillet, sauté chopped spinach and cherry tomatoes until wilted.

4. Poach the egg in simmering water until the whites are set but the yolk is still runny. Assemble the bowl by placing cooked quinoa at the bottom, followed by sautéed spinach and tomatoes, and top with the poached egg. Season with salt and pepper to taste.

Nutritional value: This breakfast is packed with protein, fiber, vitamins, and minerals. Quinoa provides essential amino acids, while spinach and tomatoes add vitamins A and C. The egg contributes additional protein and healthy fats.

Cooking time: Approximately 20-25 minutes.

8. Cottage cheese and fruit bowl with sliced almonds and a drizzle of honey:

Ingredients:

*   1/2 cup cottage cheese
*   1/2 cup mixed fruits (such as berries, banana slices, and kiwi)
*   1 tablespoon sliced almonds

- 1 teaspoon honey

Preparation:

1. Place cottage cheese in a bowl.
2. Top with mixed fruits and sliced almonds.
3. Drizzle honey over the top.
4. Optionally, sprinkle with a pinch of cinnamon or nutmeg for extra flavor.

Nutritional value: This breakfast is rich in protein from the cottage cheese and healthy fats from almonds. Fruits provide vitamins, minerals, and fiber, while honey adds natural sweetness.

9. Vegetable frittata with sweet potato hash browns:

Ingredients:

- 4 eggs
- 1/4 cup milk or non-dairy milk
- 1/2 cup diced vegetables (such as bell peppers, onions, and spinach)
- 1 medium sweet potato, grated
- Salt and pepper to taste Olive oil for cooking

Preparation:

1. Preheat the oven to 350°F (175°C).
2. In a mixing bowl, combine eggs, milk, salt, and pepper.
3. Heat the olive oil in an oven-safe skillet over medium heat. Add diced vegetables and sauté until softened.
4. Pour the egg mixture over the vegetables in the skillet.
5. Place the skillet in the preheated oven and bake for about 15-20 minutes or until the frittata is set.

6. Meanwhile, prepare sweet potato hash browns by mixing grated sweet potato with salt and pepper. Cook in a skillet with olive oil until crispy.

Nutritional value: This breakfast provides a good balance of protein, carbohydrates, and fiber. Eggs are a great source of protein and essential nutrients, while vegetables and sweet potatoes offer vitamins, minerals, and fiber.

Cooking time: Approximately 25-30 minutes.

10. Buckwheat porridge topped with cinnamon, apples, and pecans

Ingredients:

- 1/2 cup buckwheat groats
- 1 cup of milk or water (dairy or nondairy)
- 1/2 teaspoon cinnamon
- small apple, diced
- tablespoons chopped pecans
- Optional: maple syrup or honey for sweetness

Preparation:

1. Rinse the buckwheat groats under cold water.
2. Heat water or milk in a small pot until it boils. Add buckwheat groats and reduce heat to low.
3. Simmer for about 10-12 minutes or until the groats are tender and the liquid is absorbed.
4. Stir in cinnamon and diced apple.
5. Serve the porridge in bowls and top with chopped pecans. Drizzle with maple syrup or honey if desired.

Nutritional value: Buckwheat is a gluten-free whole grain rich in fiber, protein, and essential nutrients. Apples provide vitamins and antioxidants, while pecans offer healthy fats and additional protein.

Cooking time: Approximately 15 minutes.

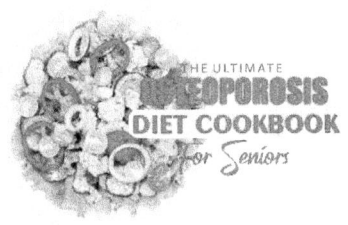

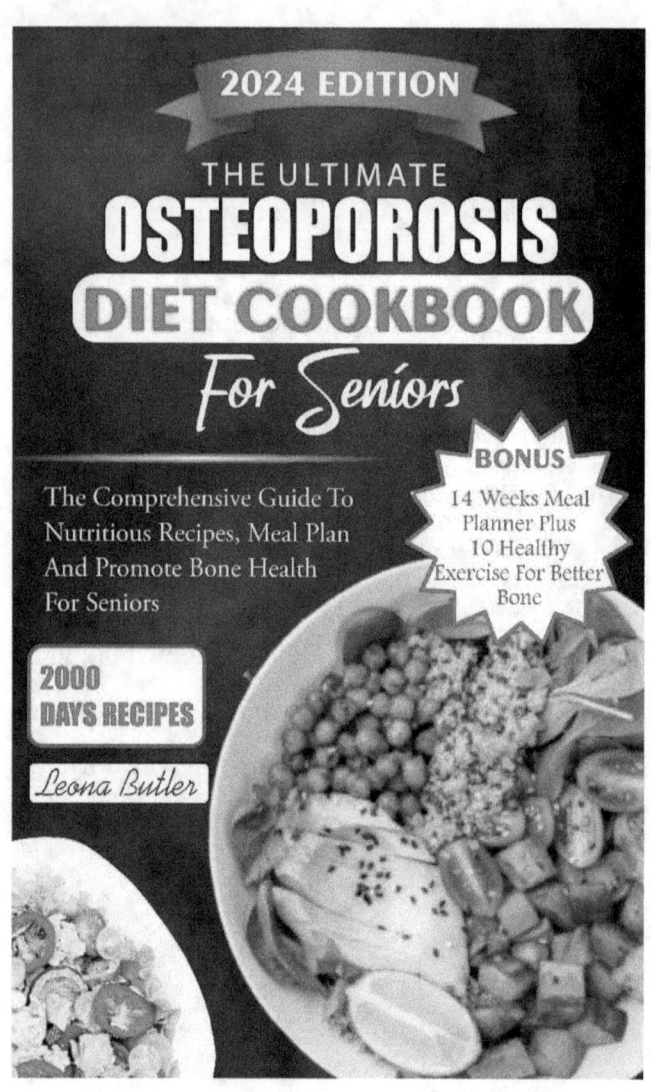

2024 EDITION

THE ULTIMATE

OSTEOPOROSIS

DIET COOKBOOK

For Seniors

The Comprehensive Guide To
Nutritious Recipes, Meal Plan
And Promote Bone Health
For Seniors

BONUS
14 Weeks Meal
Planner Plus
10 Healthy
Exercise For Better
Bone

**2000
DAYS RECIPES**

Leona Butler

Chapter 2: Lunch Recipes for

1. Grilled Chicken Salad

Ingredients:

- 200g grilled chicken breast
- 4 cups mixed greens
- 1 cup cherry tomatoes, halved
- avocado, sliced
- tbsp olive oil
- 1 tbsp balsamic vinegar Salt and pepper to taste

Preparation:

1. Season the chicken breast with salt and pepper and grill until cooked through, about 15 minutes.
2. In a large bowl, toss the mixed greens, cherry tomatoes, and avocado slices.
3. Slice the grilled chicken and add it to the salad.
4. Drizzle with olive oil and balsamic vinegar, then toss to combine.

Nutritional Value:

- Calories: ~400
- Protein: ~30g
- Carbohydrates: ~10g
- Fat: ~25g
- Fiber: ~7g

Cooking Time:

Approximately 15 minutes for grilling the chicken.

2. Quinoa and Black Bean Stuffed Peppers

Ingredients:

- 4 large bell peppers
- 1 cup quinoa
- 1 can (15 oz) of black beans, drained and rinsed
- 1 cup diced tomatoes
- 1 tsp cumin
- 1 tsp chili powder
- Salt and pepper to taste 1 cup shredded cheese (optional)

Preparation:

1. Preheat the oven to 375°F (190°C).
2. Cook quinoa according to package instructions.
3. In a large bowl, mix cooked quinoa, black beans, diced tomatoes, cumin, chili powder, salt, and pepper.
4. Cut the bell pepper tops off and remove the seeds and membranes.
5. Stuff each pepper with the quinoa mixture.
6. Place stuffed peppers in a baking dish, and if desired, sprinkle shredded cheese on top. Cover the peppers with foil and bake for 25-30 minutes, or until tender.
7. Serve with a side of steamed broccoli.

Nutritional Value:

- Calories: ~350
- Protein: ~15g
- Carbohydrates: ~55g
- Fat: ~7g
- Fiber: ~15g

Cooking Time: **25-30 minutes.**

3. Lentil Soup:

Ingredients:

- cup dried lentils
- carrots, diced
- 2 stalks celery, diced
- onion, diced
- cloves garlic, minced 1 tsp turmeric
- 6 cups vegetable broth Salt and pepper to taste

Preparation:

1. Rinse lentils under cold water and drain.
2. In a large pot, sauté onions, carrots, celery, and garlic until softened, about 5 minutes.
3. Add lentils, turmeric, vegetable broth, salt, and pepper.
4. Bring to a boil, then reduce the heat and simmer for 20-25 minutes, or until the lentils are cooked.
5. Serve hot.

Nutritional Value:

- Calories: ~250
- Protein: ~15g
- Carbohydrates: ~40g
- Fat: ~1g
- Fiber: ~15g

Cooking Time:

Approximately 25-30 minutes.

4. Tuna Salad Lettuce Wraps with Cucumber and Carrot Sticks

Ingredients:

- 2 cans of tuna (drained)
- 1/4 cup Greek yogurt
- 1 tablespoon lemon juice
- 1/4 teaspoon black pepper
- 4 large lettuce leaves
- 1 cucumber, cut into sticks 2 carrots, cut into sticks

Preparation:

1. In a bowl, combine the drained tuna, Greek yogurt, lemon juice, and black pepper. Mix well.
2. Lay out the lettuce leaves and spoon the tuna salad mixture onto each leaf. Roll up the lettuce leaves to make wraps.
3. Serve with cucumber and carrot sticks on the side. Nutritional Value:
4. High in protein from tuna and Greek yogurt.
5. Low in carbohydrates.
6. Rich in vitamins and minerals from vegetables.

Cooking Time: 10 minutes

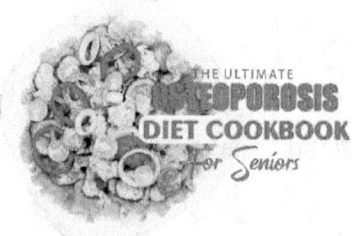

5. Roasted Vegetable Quinoa Salad with Balsamic Vinaigrette

Ingredients:

- cup quinoa
- cups water or vegetable broth
- 2 cups mixed vegetables (such as bell peppers, zucchini, and cherry tomatoes)
- 2 tablespoons olive oil
- Salt and pepper to taste
- 2 tablespoons balsamic vinegar
- 1 tablespoon honey 1 clove garlic, minced

Preparation:

1. Preheat the oven to 400°F (200°C).
2. Rinse the quinoa under cold water. In a saucepan, combine quinoa and water or broth. Bring to a boil, then reduce heat, cover, and simmer for 15 minutes or until quinoa is cooked and liquid is absorbed.

3. Meanwhile, toss the mixed vegetables with olive oil, salt, and pepper on a baking sheet. Roast the vegetables in a warm oven for 20-25 minutes, or until they are soft and slightly browned.

4. In a small bowl, whisk together balsamic vinegar, honey, minced garlic, salt, and pepper to make the vinaigrette.

5. In a large bowl, combine cooked quinoa, roasted vegetables, and balsamic vinaigrette. Mix well.

Nutritional Value:

High in fiber and protein from quinoa and vegetables. Provides essential vitamins and minerals. Heart-healthy fats from olive oil.

Cooking Time: 40-45 minutes

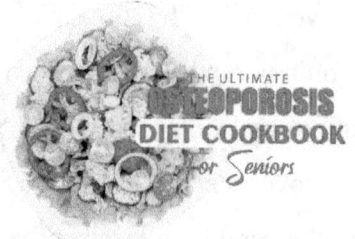

6. Salmon and Avocado Sushi Rolls with Miso Soup

Ingredients:

- 2 nori seaweed sheets
- 1 cup cooked sushi rice
- 1/2 avocado, sliced
- 4 ounces cooked salmon, flaked
- Soy sauce for dipping
- 2 cups dashi broth (can be made with instant dashi powder)
- 2 tablespoons miso paste
- 2 green onions, thinly sliced
- 1/2 cup tofu, diced (optional)
- 1 tablespoon seaweed (such as wakame), rehydrated (optional)

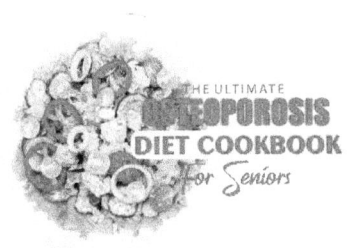

Preparation:

1. Arrange a nori sheet on a bamboo sushi mat.. Spread half of the sushi rice evenly over the nori, leaving a small border at the top.
2. Place avocado slices and salmon along the center of the rice.
3. Roll the sushi tightly using the bamboo mat. Repeat with the remaining nori, rice, avocado, and salmon.
4. Slice each roll into 6-8 pieces using a sharp knife.
5. Serve with soy sauce for dipping. For Miso Soup:
6. Heat the dashi broth in a saucepan until it simmers.
7. In a small bowl, dissolve miso paste in a ladleful of hot broth, then return the mixture to the saucepan.
8. Add green onions, tofu, and rehydrated seaweed (if using).
9. Simmer for a few minutes until thoroughly heated.

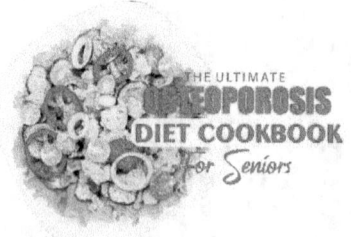

Nutritional Value:

- Rich in omega-3 fatty acids from salmon and avocado.
- Provides protein from salmon and tofu (if using).
- Low in calories and high in nutrients. Contains probiotics from miso paste.

Cooking Time: 30-35 minutes (including prep time for sushi rolls)

7. Turkey and Vegetable Stir-Fry with Brown Rice:

Ingredients:

- lb (450g) turkey breast, thinly sliced
- cups (400g) mixed vegetables (bell peppers, broccoli, carrots, snap peas)
- 2 cloves garlic, minced
- tablespoon (15ml) olive oil
- 1/4 cup (60ml) low-sodium soy sauce
- cups (400g) cooked brown rice

Preparation:

1. In a large skillet, heat the olive oil on medium-high.
2. Add minced garlic and sliced turkey breast. Cook until turkey is browned.
3. Add mixed vegetables and cook until they are tender-crisp.
4. Pour soy sauce over the turkey and vegetables, stirring well to combine.
5. Serve stir-fry over cooked brown rice.

Nutritional Value:

- Approximate Calories: 400 per serving
- Protein: 30g
- Carbohydrates: 40g
- Fat: 12g

Cooking Time: 20 minutes

8. Chickpea and Vegetable Curry served over Cauliflower Rice

Ingredients:

- can (15 oz or 425g) chickpeas, drained and rinsed
- cups (400g) mixed vegetables (such as cauliflower, carrots, bell peppers)
- onion, diced
- cloves garlic, minced
- 1 tablespoon (15ml) curry powder
- 1 can of coconut milk (13.5 oz or 400ml)
- Salt and pepper to taste 4 cups (800g) cauliflower rice

Preparation:

1. In a large skillet, sauté diced onion and minced garlic until translucent.
2. Add mixed vegetables and chickpeas, cooking until slightly tender.
3. Stir in curry powder and coconut milk. Simmer until vegetables are cooked through and sauce has thickened.

4. Season with salt and pepper to taste.

5. Serve curry over cauliflower rice.

Nutritional Value:

- Approximate Calories: 350 per serving
- Protein: 12g
- Carbohydrates: 30g
- Fat: 20g

Cooking Time: 25 minutes

9. Whole Wheat Wrap filled with Hummus, Grilled Vegetables, and Feta Cheese:

Ingredients:

- 4 whole wheat wraps
- cup (240g) hummus
- cups (400g) mixed grilled vegetables (zucchini, eggplant, bell peppers)
- 1/2 cup (75g) crumbled feta cheese

Preparation:

- Spread hummus evenly on each whole wheat wrap.
- Top with grilled vegetables and crumbled feta cheese.
- Roll the wrappers tightly, fastening them with toothpicks as needed.

Nutritional Value:

- Approximate Calories: 300 per serving
- Protein: 10g
- Carbohydrates: 35g
- Fat: 15g

Cooking Time: 15 minutes (for grilling vegetables)

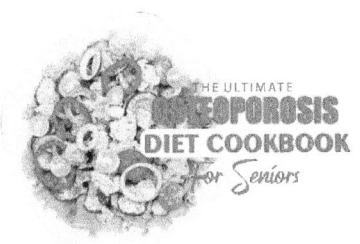

10. Minestrone Soup with Whole Grain Bread and a Side of Mixed Green Salad:

Ingredients:

- 4 cups (1 liter) vegetable broth
- 1 can (15 oz or 425g) diced tomatoes
- cup (200g) cooked small pasta (such as ditalini or small shells)
- cups (400g) mixed vegetables (carrots, celery, zucchini, green beans)
- can (15 oz or 425g) kidney beans, drained and rinsed
- cloves garlic, minced
- 1 teaspoon (5ml) dried basil
- Salt and pepper to taste
- Whole grain bread for serving
- Mixed greens for salad Balsamic vinaigrette for salad

Preparation:

1. In a large pot, combine vegetable broth, diced tomatoes, mixed vegetables, kidney beans, minced garlic, and dried basil. Bring to a boil.
2. Reduce heat and let simmer for about 20 minutes, or until vegetables are tender. Season with salt and pepper, then stir in the cooked pasta.
3. Serve hot with whole grain bread and a side of mixed green salad tossed in balsamic vinaigrette.

Nutritional Value:
- Approximate Calories: 350 per serving (soup only)
- Protein: 12g
- Carbohydrates: 60g
- Fat: 5g

Cooking Time: 30 minutes Enjoy your meals!

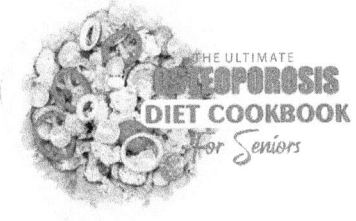

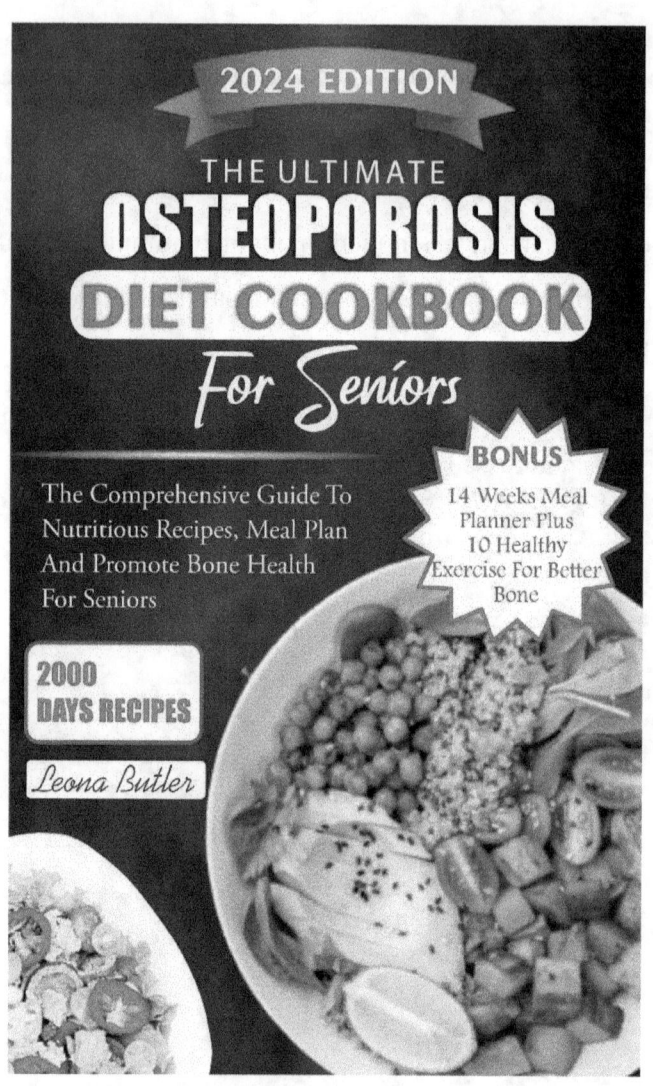

1. Baked Salmon with Roasted Brussels Sprouts and Quinoa Pilaf

Ingredients:

- Salmon: 4 fillets (6 oz each)
- Brussels Sprouts: 1 lb, trimmed and halved
- Quinoa: 1 cup, rinsed
- Vegetable Broth: 2 cups Olive Oil: 3 tbsp
- Garlic: 3 cloves, minced
- Lemon: 1, sliced
- Salt: 1 tsp
- Black Pepper: 1/2 tsp
- Paprika: 1/2 tsp
- Fresh Parsley: 2 tbsp, chopped

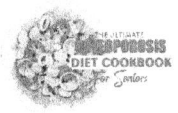

Preparation:

1. Preheat the oven to 400°F (200°C).
2. In a large baking dish, place the salmon fillets and Brussels sprouts. Drizzle with 2 tbsp of olive oil, minced garlic, salt, black pepper, and paprika. Toss to coat evenly. Arrange lemon slices over the salmon fillets.
3. Bake in the preheated oven for 15-20 minutes, or until the salmon is cooked through and Brussels sprouts are tender and slightly crispy.
4. Meanwhile, in a saucepan, heat the vegetable broth to a boil. Add quinoa, reduce heat, cover, and simmer for 15-20 minutes, or until quinoa is cooked and liquid is absorbed.
5. Fluff quinoa with a fork and stir in chopped parsley.
6. Serve baked salmon with roasted Brussels sprouts and quinoa pilaf.
7. If preferred, garnish with more lemon slices and parsley.

Nutritional Value:
- Calories: 450 per serving
- Protein: 35g

- Carbohydrates: 30g
- Fat: 20g
- Fiber: 6g

Cooking Time:

Approximately 30-40 minutes

2. Turkey Meatballs with Marinara Sauce served over Spaghetti Squash

Ingredients:

- Ground Turkey: 1 lb
- Egg: 1
- Breadcrumbs: 1/2 cup
- Parmesan Cheese: 1/4 cup, grated
- Garlic Powder: 1 tsp
- Onion Powder: 1 tsp
- Salt: 1/2 tsp
- Black Pepper: 1/2 tsp
- Olive Oil: 2 tbsp
- Spaghetti Squash: 2 medium, halved and seeded

Marinara Sauce: 2 cups Fresh Basil: for garnish

Preparation:

1. Preheat the oven to 400°F (200°C).
2. In a large bowl, combine ground turkey, egg, breadcrumbs, Parmesan cheese, garlic powder, onion powder, salt, and black pepper. Mix until well combined.
3. Shape the mixture into meatballs (approximately 1.5 inches in diameter).
4. In a large skillet, heat the olive oil over medium heat. Cook the meatballs until browned on all sides, which should take about 5-7 minutes.
5. Transfer the meatballs to a baking dish and pour marinara sauce over them.
6. Place the halved spaghetti squash on a baking sheet, cut side down. Bake both the meatballs and spaghetti squash in the preheated oven for 25-30 minutes, or until squash is tender. With a fork, scrape the spaghetti squash into strands.
7. Serve the turkey meatballs with marinara sauce over spaghetti squash strands. Garnish with fresh basil.

Nutritional Value:

- Calories: 380 per serving
- Protein: 30g
- Carbohydrates: 25g
- Fat: 15g
- Fiber: 5g

Cooking Time:

Approximately 40-45 minutes

3. Grilled Tofu and Vegetable Kebabs with Quinoa Tabbouleh

Ingredients:

- Extra Firm Tofu: 1 block (14 oz), pressed and cut into cubes
- Bell Peppers: 2, assorted colors, cut into chunks
- Zucchini: 2, sliced
- Red Onion: 1, cut into chunks
- Cherry Tomatoes: 1 cup Quinoa: 1 cup, rinsed

- Vegetable Broth: 2 cups
- Cucumber: 1, diced
- Fresh Parsley: 1/4 cup, chopped
- Fresh Mint: 2 tbsp, chopped
- Lemon Juice: 2 tbsp
- Olive Oil: 2 tbsp
- Salt: 1/2 tsp
- Black Pepper: 1/4 tsp Skewers: for assembling kebabs

Preparation:

1. Preheat the grill to medium-high heat.
2. Thread tofu cubes, bell peppers, zucchini, red onion, and cherry tomatoes onto skewers, alternating between ingredients.
3. Heat vegetable broth in a saucepan.. Add quinoa, reduce heat, cover, and simmer for 15-20 minutes, or until quinoa is cooked and liquid is absorbed.
4. In a large bowl, combine cooked quinoa, diced cucumber, chopped parsley, chopped mint, lemon juice, olive oil, salt, and black pepper. Mix well to combine.

5. Grill the tofu and vegetable kebabs for 10-12 minutes, turning occasionally, until vegetables are tender and lightly charred.

6. Serve grilled tofu and vegetable kebabs with quinoa tabbouleh.

Nutritional Value:

- Calories: 320 per serving
- Protein: 15g
- Carbohydrates: 35g
- Fat: 15g
- Fiber: 8g

Cooking Time:

Approximately 25-30 minutes

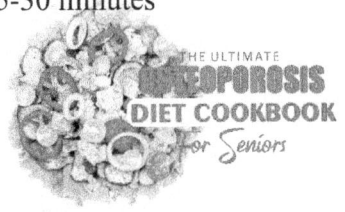

4. Beef and Broccoli Stir-Fry with Brown Rice:

Ingredients:

- lb (450g) beef sirloin, thinly sliced
- cups broccoli florets
- 2 tablespoons soy sauce
- 1 tablespoon oyster sauce
- tablespoon cornstarch
- cloves garlic, minced
- tablespoon vegetable oil
- cups cooked brown rice

Preparation:

1. In a bowl, combine the soy sauce, oyster sauce, and cornstarch. Marinate sliced beef for 15 minutes.
2. In a skillet, heat the vegetable oil on medium-high. Add the minced garlic and sauté until fragrant.
3. Add marinated beef to the skillet and stir-fry until browned, about 2-3 minutes.

4. Add broccoli florets and continue to stir-fry until they are tender-crisp, about 4-5 minutes. Serve the stir-fry over cooked brown rice.

Nutritional Value:

This dish is high in protein from the beef and broccoli.

Brown rice adds fiber and complex carbohydrates.

Each serving provides approximately 400-500 calories.

Cooking Time:

Total cooking time: 20-25 minutes.

5. Stuffed Acorn Squash with Ground Turkey, Quinoa, and Cranberries:

Ingredients:

- 2 acorn squashes, halved and seeds removed
- 1 lb (450g) ground turkey
- 1 cup cooked quinoa
- 1/2 cup dried cranberries
- 1 teaspoon ground cinnamon

- Salt and pepper to taste Olive oil for drizzling

Preparation:

1. Preheat the oven to 375°F (190°C).
2. Drizzle the insides of the acorn squash halves with olive oil and season with salt and pepper.
3. Place them cut side down on a baking sheet and roast for 25 minutes.
4. In a skillet, cook ground turkey until browned. Drain any excess fat.
5. In a bowl, mix cooked quinoa, dried cranberries, ground cinnamon, and cooked ground turkey.
6. Stuff the roasted acorn squash halves with the turkey-quinoa mixture.
7. Return stuffed squash to the oven and bake for an additional 15-20 minutes, until squash is tender.

Nutritional Value:

- This dish is rich in protein from the turkey and quinoa.
- Acorn squash provides vitamins and minerals, while cranberries add a touch of sweetness. Each serving provides approximately 350-400 calories.

Cooking Time:

Total cooking time: 45-50 minutes.

6. Vegetable Lasagna made with Whole Wheat Noodles and Ricotta Cheese:

Ingredients:

- 9 whole wheat lasagna noodles
- 2 cups marinara sauce
- 2 cups chopped mixed veggies (such as mushrooms, zucchini, and bell peppers)
- 1 cup part-skim ricotta cheese
- 1 cup shredded mozzarella cheese
- 1/4 cup grated Parmesan cheese
- 1 teaspoon dried basil Salt and pepper to taste

Preparation:

1. Preheat the oven to 375°F (190°C).
2. Cook the lasagna noodles according to package directions, then drain and put aside. In a bowl, combine the chopped veggies, ricotta cheese, shredded mozzarella cheese, dried basil, salt, and pepper.
3. Spread a thin layer of marinara sauce in the bottom of a 9x13-inch baking dish. Layer three cooked lasagna noodles on top of the sauce.
4. Spread half of the vegetable-ricotta mixture over the noodles.
5. Repeat layers with marinara sauce, noodles, and the remaining vegetable-ricotta mixture. Top with the remaining marinara sauce and sprinkle with grated Parmesan cheese.
6. Bake for 30 minutes with the dish covered with foil. Then, remove the foil and bake for an additional 15 minutes, until cheese is bubbly and golden.

Nutritional Value:

- This dish is high in fiber from the whole wheat noodles and vegetables.

- Ricotta cheese provides protein and calcium.

- Each serving provides approximately 300-350 calories.

Cooking Time:

Total cooking time: 1 hour 15 minutes.

7. Baked Chicken Breast with Sweet Potato Mash and Steamed Green Beans

Ingredients:

- 2 chicken breasts (about 8 oz each)
- 2 medium sweet potatoes
- 1 cup green beans
- Olive oil
- Salt and pepper to taste

Preparation:

1. Preheat oven to 375°F (190°C).
2. Season chicken breasts with salt and pepper, drizzle with olive oil, and place on a baking sheet.
3. Bake chicken breasts for 25-30 minutes or until cooked through.
4. Peel and dice sweet potatoes, then boil them until tender.
5. Drain sweet potatoes and mash them with a fork or potato masher.
6. Steam green beans until tender.
7. Serve baked chicken breasts with sweet potato mash and steamed green beans.

Nutritional Value:

- Chicken breasts: High in protein and low in fat
- Sweet potatoes: Rich in vitamins A and C, fiber
- Green beans: Low in calories, high in fiber and vitamins

Cooking Time: 30-35 minutes

8. Lentil and Vegetable Stew served with a Side of Whole Grain Bread

Ingredients:

- cup lentils
- carrots, diced
- 2 celery stalks, diced
- onion, chopped
- cloves garlic, minced 4 cups vegetable broth
- Salt and pepper to taste Whole grain bread slices

Preparation:

1. In a large pot, cook the onions and garlic until tender.
2. Add diced carrots and celery, cook until slightly tender.
3. Rinse lentils and add them to the pot along with vegetable broth.
4. Season with salt and pepper, bring to a boil, then reduce heat and simmer for 20-25 minutes or until lentils are tender.

5. Serve the lentil and vegetable stew with slices of whole grain bread.

Nutritional Value:
- Lentils: High in protein, fiber, and various nutrients
- Vegetables: Rich in vitamins and minerals
- Whole grain bread: High in fiber and nutrients

Cooking Time: 25-30 minutes

9. Shrimp and Vegetable Stir-Fry with Sesame Ginger Sauce over Brown Rice Noodles

Ingredients:

- lb shrimp, peeled and deveined
- cups mixed vegetables (bell peppers, broccoli, carrots, etc.)
- 8 oz brown rice noodles
- 2 tablespoons sesame oil
- 2 tablespoons soy sauce
- 1 tablespoon honey

- 1 tablespoon minced ginger 2 cloves garlic, minced

Preparation:

1. Cook brown rice noodles according to package instructions.
2. Heat sesame oil in a large skillet over medium heat.
3. Add minced ginger and garlic, sauté until fragrant.
4. Add shrimp and mixed vegetables, stir-fry until shrimp are pink and vegetables are tender.
5. In a small bowl, mix soy sauce and honey, then pour over the shrimp and vegetables.
6. Serve the stir-fry over cooked brown rice noodles.

Nutritional Value:
- Shrimp: Low in calories, high in protein
- Vegetables: Rich in vitamins and minerals
- Brown rice noodles: Whole grain option, high in fiber

Cooking Time: 20-25 minutes

10. Roasted Cauliflower Steaks with Tahini Sauce and a Side of Wild Rice Pilaf

Ingredients:

- head cauliflower
- tablespoons olive oil
- Salt and pepper to taste
- ½ cup tahini
- 2 tablespoons lemon juice
- cup wild rice
- cups water or vegetable broth Fresh parsley for garnish

Preparation:

1. Preheat oven to 425°F (220°C).
2. Slice cauliflower into thick "steaks", drizzle with olive oil, and season with salt and pepper.
3. Roast cauliflower steaks in the oven for 25-30 minutes or until tender and golden brown.
4. In a small bowl, whisk together tahini, lemon juice, and a splash of water until smooth. Cook wild rice according

to package instructions, using water or vegetable broth for added flavor.

5. Serve roasted cauliflower steaks with tahini sauce drizzled on top and a side of wild rice pilaf. Garnish with fresh parsley.

Nutritional Value:

- Cauliflower: Low in calories, high in fiber and vitamins
- Tahini: Good source of healthy fats and protein
- Wild rice: Nutrient-dense, high in fiber

Cooking Time: 30-35 minutes

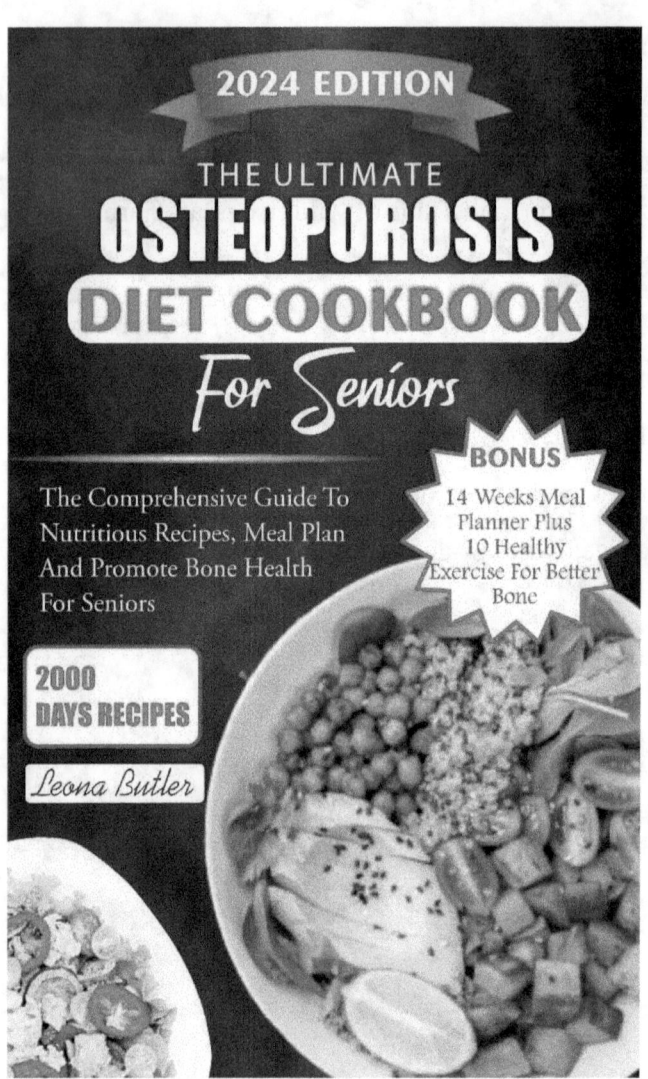

2024 EDITION

THE ULTIMATE

OSTEOPOROSIS

DIET COOKBOOK

For Seniors

The Comprehensive Guide To
Nutritious Recipes, Meal Plan
And Promote Bone Health
For Seniors

BONUS
14 Weeks Meal
Planner Plus
10 Healthy
Exercise For Better
Bone

**2000
DAYS RECIPES**

Leona Butler

Chapter 4: Snacks and Desserts for Bone Support:

1. Almond Butter and Banana Slices on Whole Grain Crackers

Ingredients:

- Whole grain crackers: 8 pieces
- Almond butter: 4 tablespoons Banana: 1, sliced

Preparation:

1. Spread ½ tablespoon of almond butter on each whole grain cracker.
2. Top each cracker with banana slices.

Nutritional Value (per serving):

- Calories: 240
- Protein: 5g
- Carbohydrates: 35g
- Fiber: 6g
- Fat: 10g

- Sugars: 10g

Cooking Time:

Preparation Time: 5 minutes

2. Greek Yogurt with Honey and Sliced Almonds

Ingredients:

- Greek yogurt: 1 cup
- Honey: 2 tablespoons Sliced almonds: 2 tablespoons

Preparation:
- Spoon the Greek yogurt into a bowl.
- Drizzle honey over the yogurt.
- Sprinkle sliced almonds on top.

Nutritional Value (per serving):
- Calories: 290
- Protein: 18g
- Carbohydrates: 27g
- Fiber: 2g

- Fat: 13g
- Sugars: 22g

Cooking Time:

Preparation Time: 3 minutes

3. Apple Slices with Almond Butter and Cinnamon

Ingredients:

- Apple: 1, sliced
- Almond butter: 2 tablespoons
- Cinnamon: ¼ teaspoon

Preparation:

- Spread almond butter on apple slices.
- Sprinkle cinnamon over the almond butter.

Nutritional Value (per serving):

- Calories: 210
- Protein: 4g

- Carbohydrates: 25g
- Fiber: 7g
- Fat: 12g
- Sugars: 15g

Cooking Time:
Preparation Time: 2 minutes

4. Carrot and Hummus Snack Packs

Ingredients:

- 2 medium carrots, peeled and cut into sticks
- 1/2 cup hummus
- Optional: celery sticks, cucumber slices

Preparation:

1. Wash and peel the carrots, then cut them into sticks.
2. Portion out the hummus into individual snack-sized containers.

3. Place the carrot sticks alongside the hummus in the containers.

4. Optionally, include celery sticks or cucumber slices for variety.

Nutritional Value:

- Carrots are rich in vitamin A, fiber, and antioxidants.

- Hummus provides protein, fiber, and healthy fats.

- This snack is low in calories yet great in nutrition.

5. Trail Mix with Almonds, Dried Cranberries, and Pumpkin Seeds:

Ingredients:

- 1/2 cup almonds
- 1/4 cup dried cranberries
- 1/4 cup pumpkin seeds

Preparation:

1. Measure out the almonds, dried cranberries, and pumpkin seeds. Mix all ingredients together in a bowl until evenly distributed.
2. Divide the trail mix into individual snack-sized portions or store in an airtight container.

Nutritional Value:

- Almonds provide protein, good fats, and vitamin E.
- Dried cranberries add natural sweetness and antioxidants.
- Pumpkin seeds are a good source of protein, iron, and magnesium.

6. Cottage Cheese with Pineapple Chunks and Sunflower Seeds

Ingredients:

- 1/2 cup cottage cheese
- 1/2 cup diced pineapple (fresh or canned, drained)
- 2 tablespoons sunflower seeds

Preparation:

1. Measure out the cottage cheese, pineapple chunks, and sunflower seeds.
2. Combine cottage cheese and pineapple chunks in a bowl.
3. Sprinkle sunflower seeds on top.

Nutritional Value:

- Cottage cheese is rich in protein and calcium.
- Pineapple provides vitamin C and bromelain, an enzyme with anti-inflammatory properties. Sunflower seeds include healthful lipids, protein, and vitamin E.

7. Dark Chocolate Covered Strawberries:

Ingredients:

- 1 pound of fresh strawberries
- 8 ounces of dark chocolate (at least 70% cocoa)

Preparation:

1. Wash and dry the strawberries thoroughly.

2. Melt the dark chocolate in a microwave-safe bowl, stirring every 30 seconds until smooth.
3. Dip each strawberry into the melted chocolate, coating it halfway.
4. Place the chocolate-covered strawberries on a parchment-lined baking sheet.
5. Refrigerate for about 30 minutes or until the chocolate sets.

Nutritional Value: Dark chocolate provides antioxidants and may improve heart health when consumed in moderation.

Cooking Time: Approximately 30 minutes.

8. Baked Apple Chips Sprinkled with Cinnamon:

Ingredients:

- 2 large apples
- 1 teaspoon of ground cinnamon

Preparation:

1. Preheat the oven to 200°F (93°C).
2. Slice the apples thinly, about 1/8 inch thick, and remove any seeds.
3. Place the apple slices on a baking sheet covered with parchment paper.
4. Sprinkle the cinnamon evenly over the apple slices.
5. Bake for 1.5 to 2 hours, flipping the slices halfway through, until they are crispy and golden brown.

Nutritional Value: Apples are a good source of fiber and vitamin C, while cinnamon may help regulate blood sugar levels.

Cooking Time: Approximately 1.5 to 2 hours.

9. Chia Seed Pudding with Mixed Berries

Ingredients:

- 1/4 cup of chia seeds
- 1 cup almond milk (or other milk of your choosing)
- 1 tablespoon of honey (optional) Mixed berries for topping

Preparation:

1. In a bowl, mix together the chia seeds, almond milk, and honey (if using).
2. Let the mixture sit for at least 2 hours, or preferably overnight, in the refrigerator, stirring occasionally until it thickens into a pudding-like consistency.
3. Serve the chia seed pudding topped with mixed berries.

Nutritional Value: Chia seeds are rich in fiber, protein, and omega-3 fatty acids, while berries provide antioxidants and vitamins.

Cooking Time: Approximately 2 hours or overnight for soaking.

10. Frozen Yogurt Bark with Chopped Nuts and Dried Fruit

Ingredients:

- 2 cups of Greek yogurt
- 1/4 cup chopped nuts (almonds or walnuts) 1/4 cup of dried fruit (such as cranberries or raisins)

Preparation:

1. Line a baking sheet with parchment paper.
2. Spread the Greek yogurt evenly onto the parchment paper, about 1/4 inch thick.
3. Sprinkle the chopped nuts and dried fruit over the yogurt.
4. Place the baking sheet in the freezer for at least 2 hours, or until the yogurt is completely frozen.
5. Once frozen, break the yogurt bark into pieces and serve immediately.

Nutritional Value: Greek yogurt is high in protein and probiotics, while nuts and dried fruit provide healthy fats and fiber.

Cooking Time: Approximately 2 hours for freezing.

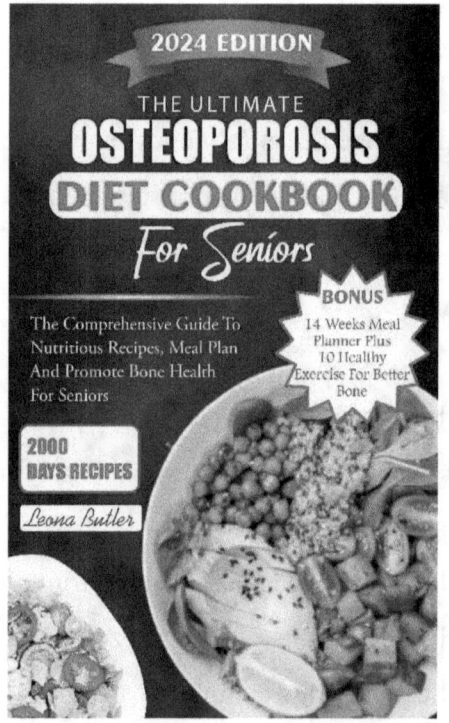

Chapter 6: 14-day meal plan

Day 1:

- Breakfast: Greek yogurt parfait with mixed berries and almond slices
- Lunch: Lentil soup with carrots, celery, and turmeric
- Dinner: Baked salmon with roasted Brussels sprouts and quinoa pilaf
- Snack/Dessert: Almond butter and banana slices on whole grain crackers

Day 2:

- Breakfast: Overnight oats with chia seeds, chopped nuts, and dried apricots
- Lunch: Turkey and vegetable stir-fry with brown rice
- Dinner: Turkey meatballs with marinara sauce served over spaghetti squash
- Snack/Dessert: Greek yogurt with honey and sliced almonds

DAY 3

- Breakfast: Avocado toast with smoked salmon and poached egg
- Lunch: Grilled chicken salad with mixed greens, cherry tomatoes, and avocado
- Dinner: Grilled tofu and vegetable kebabs with quinoa tabbouleh
- Snack/Dessert: Apple slices with almond butter and cinnamon

Day 4:

- Breakfast: Whole grain pancakes with mashed banana and walnuts
- Lunch: Chickpea and vegetable curry served over cauliflower rice
- Dinner: Beef and broccoli stir-fry with brown rice
  Snack/Dessert: Carrot and hummus snack packs

Day 5:

- Breakfast: Smoothie made with kale, pineapple, Greek yogurt, and hemp seeds
- Lunch: Whole wheat wrap filled with hummus, grilled vegetables, and feta cheese
- Dinner: Stuffed acorn squash with ground turkey, quinoa, and cranberries
- Snack/Dessert: Trail mix with almonds, dried cranberries, and pumpkin seeds

Day 6:

- Breakfast: Quinoa breakfast bowl with sautéed spinach, tomatoes, and a poached egg
- Lunch: Minestrone soup with whole grain bread and a side of mixed green salad
- Dinner: Vegetable lasagna made with whole wheat noodles and ricotta cheese
- Snack/Dessert: Cottage cheese with pineapple chunks and sunflower seeds

Day 7:

- Breakfast: Spinach and feta omelette with whole grain toast
- Lunch: Salmon and avocado sushi rolls with miso soup
- Dinner: Baked chicken breast with sweet potato mash and steamed green beans
- Snack/Dessert: Dark chocolate covered strawberries

Day 8:

- Breakfast: Greek yogurt parfait with mixed berries and almond slices
- Lunch: Lentil soup with carrots, celery, and turmeric
- Dinner: Baked salmon with roasted Brussels sprouts and quinoa pilaf
- Snack/Dessert: Almond butter and banana slices on whole grain crackers

Day 9:

- Breakfast: Overnight oats with chia seeds, chopped nuts, and dried apricots
- Lunch: Turkey and vegetable stir-fry with brown rice
- Dinner: Turkey meatballs with marinara sauce served over spaghetti squash
- Snack/Dessert: Greek yogurt with honey and sliced almonds

Day 10:

- Breakfast: Avocado toast with smoked salmon and poached egg
- Lunch: Grilled chicken salad with mixed greens, cherry tomatoes, and avocado
- Dinner: Grilled tofu and vegetable kebabs with quinoa tabbouleh
- Snack/Dessert: Apple slices with almond butter and cinnamon

Day 11:

- Breakfast: Whole grain pancakes with mashed banana and walnuts
- Lunch: Chickpea and vegetable curry served over cauliflower rice
- Dinner: Beef and broccoli stir-fry with brown rice
- Snack/Dessert: Carrot and hummus snack packs

Day 12:

- Breakfast: Smoothie made with kale, pineapple, Greek yogurt, and hemp seeds
- Lunch: Whole wheat wrap filled with hummus, grilled vegetables, and feta cheese
- Dinner: Stuffed acorn squash with ground turkey, quinoa, and cranberries
- Snack/Dessert: Trail mix with almonds, dried cranberries, and pumpkin seeds

Day 13:

- Breakfast: Quinoa breakfast bowl with sautéed spinach, tomatoes, and a poached egg
- Lunch: Minestrone soup with whole grain bread and a side of mixed green salad
- Dinner: Vegetable lasagna made with whole wheat noodles and ricotta cheese
- Snack/Dessert: Cottage cheese with pineapple chunks and sunflower seeds

Day 14:

- Breakfast: Spinach and feta omelette with whole grain toast
- Lunch: Salmon and avocado sushi rolls with miso soup
- Dinner: Baked chicken breast with sweet potato mash and steamed green beans
- Snack/Dessert: Dark chocolate covered strawberries

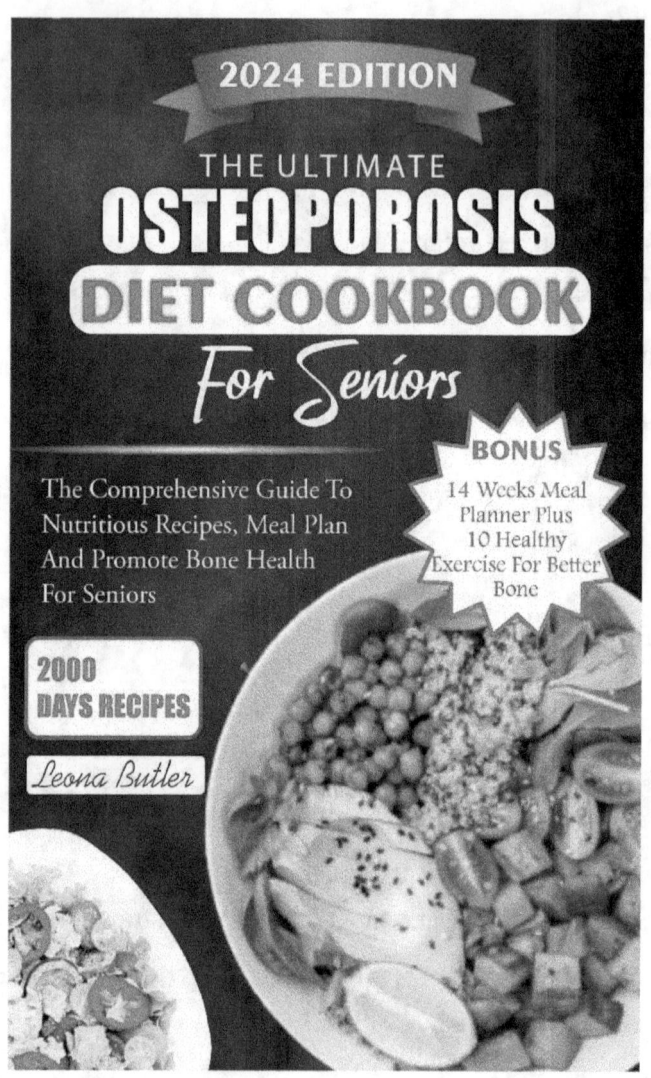

2024 EDITION

THE ULTIMATE

OSTEOPOROSIS

DIET COOKBOOK

For Seniors

The Comprehensive Guide To
Nutritious Recipes, Meal Plan
And Promote Bone Health
For Seniors

BONUS
14 Weeks Meal
Planner Plus
10 Healthy
Exercise For Better
Bone

**2000
DAYS RECIPES**

Leona Butler

1. Walking:

To perform walking exercises effectively, start by choosing comfortable footwear and suitable terrain. Begin with a gentle warm-up, then maintain proper posture with shoulders back and arms swinging naturally. Keep a steady pace, focusing on breathing deeply. Gradually increase speed or distance as endurance improves. Cool down with stretches afterward.

2. Swimming or water aerobics

To perform swimming or water aerobics effectively, start with proper warm-up exercises. In the water, maintain good posture and engage your core muscles. Gradually increase intensity by incorporating various strokes or movements. Focus on smooth, controlled motions to avoid strain. Cool down with stretches to promote flexibility and reduce muscle tension.

3. Tai chi:

To perform Tai Chi effectively, begin with a relaxed stance, feet shoulder-width apart. Keep a straight posture, chin tucked in, and shoulders relaxed. Move slowly and smoothly, coordinating breath with movement. Focus on balance, grounding, and maintaining fluidity throughout each motion, emphasizing relaxation and mindfulness. Practice regularly for optimal benefits.

4. Yoga

To perform yoga exercises perfectly, start by finding a quiet, comfortable space. Begin with deep breathing to center yourself. Gradually move through poses, focusing on proper alignment and breathing. Engage muscles and hold each pose with control. Transition smoothly between poses, maintaining balance and mindfulness throughout the practice.

5. Cycling:

To execute cycling effectively, adjust the seat height so your legs extend comfortably when pedaling. Start with a warm-up, then maintain a steady pace, engaging core muscles for stability. Focus on smooth, circular pedal strokes, breathing steadily. Gradually increase resistance for a challenge, and cool down with a gentle ride.

6. Chair exercises

To perform chair exercises effectively, sit tall with feet flat on the floor. Engage core muscles and maintain proper posture throughout. Start with gentle movements like arm raises, leg lifts, and seated marches. Gradually increase intensity and duration as strength improves. Remember to breathe deeply and stay hydrated.

7. Stretching:

To perform stretching exercises effectively, start with a gentle warm-up like walking or light jogging. Then, gradually stretch each major muscle group, holding each stretch for 15-30 seconds without bouncing. Breathe deeply and relax into each stretch, aiming for a gentle pull, not pain. Repeat the routine daily for optimal flexibility benefits.

8. Pilates:

To perform Pilates exercises effectively, focus on controlled movements, engaging your core throughout. Begin with proper alignment, breathing deeply into your ribcage. Execute each movement with precision, maintaining stability and fluidity. Emphasize control over speed, aiming for smooth transitions. Gradually progress in difficulty, ensuring mindful awareness of your body.

9. Low-impact aerobics:

To perform low-impact aerobics effectively, start with a gentle warm-up like marching in place. Then, incorporate movements such as side steps, arm raises, and knee lifts, maintaining a steady pace throughout. Focus on maintaining good posture, engaging core muscles, and breathing deeply. Cool down with light stretches afterwards to prevent stiffness.

10. Resistance band exercises

To perform resistance band exercises effectively, start with proper band selection based on resistance level. Securely anchor the band, ensuring it won't snap back. Maintain proper form throughout each movement, controlling both the extension and contraction phases. Gradually increase resistance for progressive strength gains. Always prioritize safety and consistency in your routine.

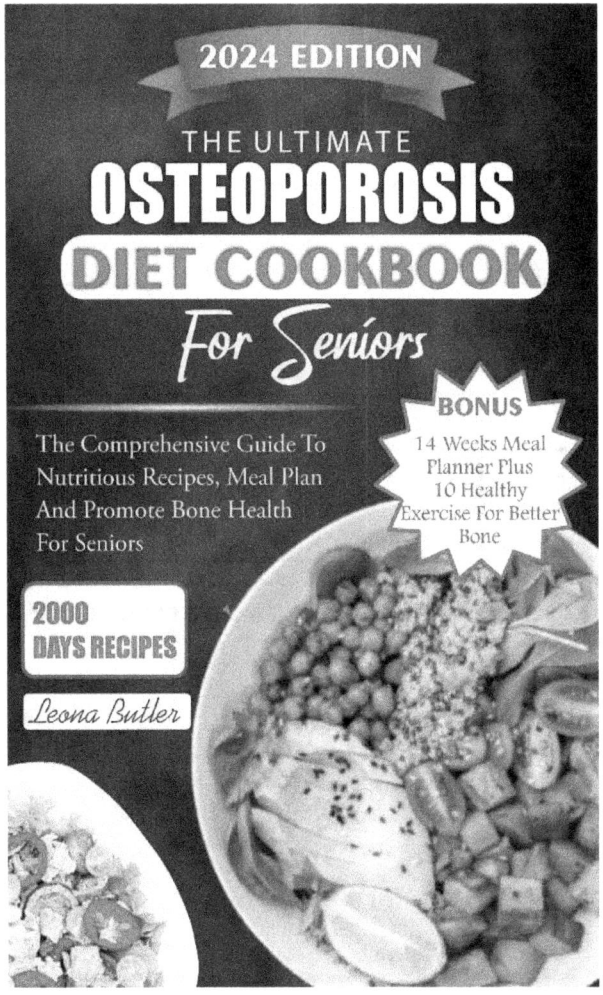

BONUS 2: 14 weeks meal planner

The Paperback of This Version Has a Free 14 Weeks Meal Planner

MY WEEKLY MEAL PLANNER
Date

	Breakfast	Lunch	Dinner
MON			
TUE			
WED			
THU			
FRI			
SAT			
SUN			

SHOPPING LIST:

- ....
- ....
- ....
- ....

TO DO LIST

....
....
....
....

NOTES
AND TIPS

Conclusion

In conclusion, embracing a tailored diet for osteoarthritis offers seniors a pathway to reclaiming control over their health and well-being. This cookbook serves as a beacon of empowerment, offering not just recipes but a holistic approach to managing the challenges of osteoarthritis. By prioritizing nutrient-dense foods, incorporating anti-inflammatory ingredients, and making mindful choices, seniors can experience significant improvements in their symptoms and overall quality of life. Beyond mere sustenance, each dish becomes a tool for healing and rejuvenation. As seniors embark on this culinary journey, they are equipped with the knowledge and resources to nourish their bodies, alleviate discomfort, and foster resilience. Together, let us savor the flavors of vitality, and may this cookbook be a trusted companion in the pursuit of lasting health and vitality for our beloved seniors.

MY WEEKLY MEAL PLANNER

Date

	Breakfast	Lunch	Dinner
MON			
TUE			
WED			
THU			
FRI			
SAT			
SUN			

SHOPPING LIST:

- ....
- ....
- ....
- ....

TO DO LIST

....
....
....
....

NOTES
AND TIPS

MY WEEKLY MEAL PLANNER

Date

	Breakfast	Lunch	Dinner
MON			
TUE			
WED			
THU			
FRI			
SAT			
SUN			

SHOPPING LIST:

TO DO LIST

- • ·
- • ·
- • ·
- • ·

NOTES
AND TIPS

MY WEEKLY MEAL PLANNER

Date

	Breakfast	Lunch	Dinner
MON			
TUE			
WED			
THU			
FRI			
SAT			
SUN			

SHOPPING LIST:

- ....
- ....
- ....
- ....

TO DO LIST

....
....
....
....

NOTES
AND TIPS

MY WEEKLY MEAL PLANNER

Date

	Breakfast	Lunch	Dinner
MON			
TUE			
WED			
THU			
FRI			
SAT			
SUN			

SHOPPING LIST:

- -
- -
- -
- -

TO DO LIST
- - - - - - - - - - - - - - - -
- - - - - - - - - - - - - - - -
- - - - - - - - - - - - - - - -
- - - - - - - - - - - - - - - -
- - - - - - - - - - - - - - - -

NOTES
AND TIPS

MY WEEKLY MEAL PLANNER

Date

	Breakfast	Lunch	Dinner
MON			
TUE			
WED			
THU			
FRI			
SAT			
SUN			

SHOPPING LIST:

TO DO LIST

- ....
- ....
- ....
- ....

NOTES
AND TIPS

MY WEEKLY MEAL PLANNER

Date

	Breakfast	Lunch	Dinner
MON			
TUE			
WED			
THU			
FRI			
SAT			
SUN			

SHOPPING LIST:

- • . . . .
- • . . . .
- • . . . .
- • . . . .

TO DO LIST

. . . .
. . . .
. . . .
. . . .

NOTES
AND TIPS

MY WEEKLY MEAL PLANNER

Date

	Breakfast	Lunch	Dinner
MON			
TUE			
WED			
THU			
FRI			
SAT			
SUN			

SHOPPING LIST:

- ·
- ·
- ·
- ·

TO DO LIST

· · · · · · · · · · · · · · · · ·
· · · · · · · · · · · · · · · · ·
· · · · · · · · · · · · · · · · ·
· · · · · · · · · · · · · · · · ·

NOTES
AND TIPS

MY WEEKLY MEAL PLANNER

Date

	Breakfast	Lunch	Dinner
MON			
TUE			
WED			
THU			
FRI			
SAT			
SUN			

SHOPPING LIST:

- ....
- ....
- ....
- ....

TO DO LIST

....
....
....
....
....

NOTES
AND TIPS

MY WEEKLY MEAL PLANNER

Date

	Breakfast	Lunch	Dinner
MON			
TUE			
WED			
THU			
FRI			
SAT			
SUN			

SHOPPING LIST:

- ....
- ....
- ....
- ....

TO DO LIST
....
....
....
....
....

NOTES AND TIPS

MY WEEKLY MEAL PLANNER

Date

	Breakfast	Lunch	Dinner
MON			
TUE			
WED			
THU			
FRI			
SAT			
SUN			

SHOPPING LIST:

- ·
- ·
- ·
- ·

TO DO LIST

· · · · · · · · · · · · · · · ·
· · · · · · · · · · · · · · · ·
· · · · · · · · · · · · · · · ·
· · · · · · · · · · · · · · · ·

NOTES
AND TIPS

MY WEEKLY MEAL PLANNER

Date

	Breakfast	Lunch	Dinner
MON			
TUE			
WED			
THU			
FRI			
SAT			
SUN			

SHOPPING LIST:

- ....
- ....
- ....
- ....

TO DO LIST

....
....
....
....
....

NOTES
AND TIPS

MY WEEKLY MEAL PLANNER

Date

	Breakfast	Lunch	Dinner
MON			
TUE			
WED			
THU			
FRI			
SAT			
SUN			

SHOPPING LIST:

- . . . .
- . . . .
- . . . .
- . . . .

TO DO LIST

. . . .
. . . .
. . . .
. . . .
. . . .

NOTES
AND TIPS

MY WEEKLY MEAL PLANNER

Date

	Breakfast	Lunch	Dinner
MON			
TUE			
WED			
THU			
FRI			
SAT			
SUN			

SHOPPING LIST:

TO DO LIST

- •..........................
- •..........................
- •..........................
- •..........................

NOTES
AND TIPS

MY WEEKLY MEAL PLANNER

Date

	Breakfast	Lunch	Dinner
MON			
TUE			
WED			
THU			
FRI			
SAT			
SUN			

SHOPPING LIST:

- ● . . . .
- ● . . . .
- ● . . . .
- ● . . . .

TO DO LIST
. . . .
. . . .
. . . .
. . . .
. . . .

NOTES
AND TIPS

MY WEEKLY MEAL PLANNER

Date

	Breakfast	Lunch	Dinner
MON			
TUE			
WED			
THU			
FRI			
SAT			
SUN			

SHOPPING LIST:

- ● . . . .
- ● . . . .
- ● . . . .
- ● . . . .

TO DO LIST

. . . .
. . . .
. . . .
. . . .
. . . .

NOTES
AND TIPS

www.ingramcontent.com/pod-product-compliance
Lightning Source LLC
Chambersburg PA
CBHW071051290526
45795CB00004B/1437